Workout Sex Coupons For Her

I0435461

J.L. Silver

INTRO:

Workout Sex Coupons are something that I have been doing for a couple of years with my lover. We give each other rewards for doing what we should do and achieving are fitness goals. This makes it fun. Inside I have included 8 examples of some workout sex coupons that you can try out, but that is not all. This is where it gets extra fun for you. I have also included 4 blank coupons for you and her to fill in. This will let you try out things that you will enjoy, goals that you have set, and whatever hard limits you might have on sex. I hope you enjoy and you can always just order the 50 page Workout Goals, Rewards, and Fails: Blank Sex Coupons for Her & Him. that you to fill in as well when you run out. All the best,

JL. Silver

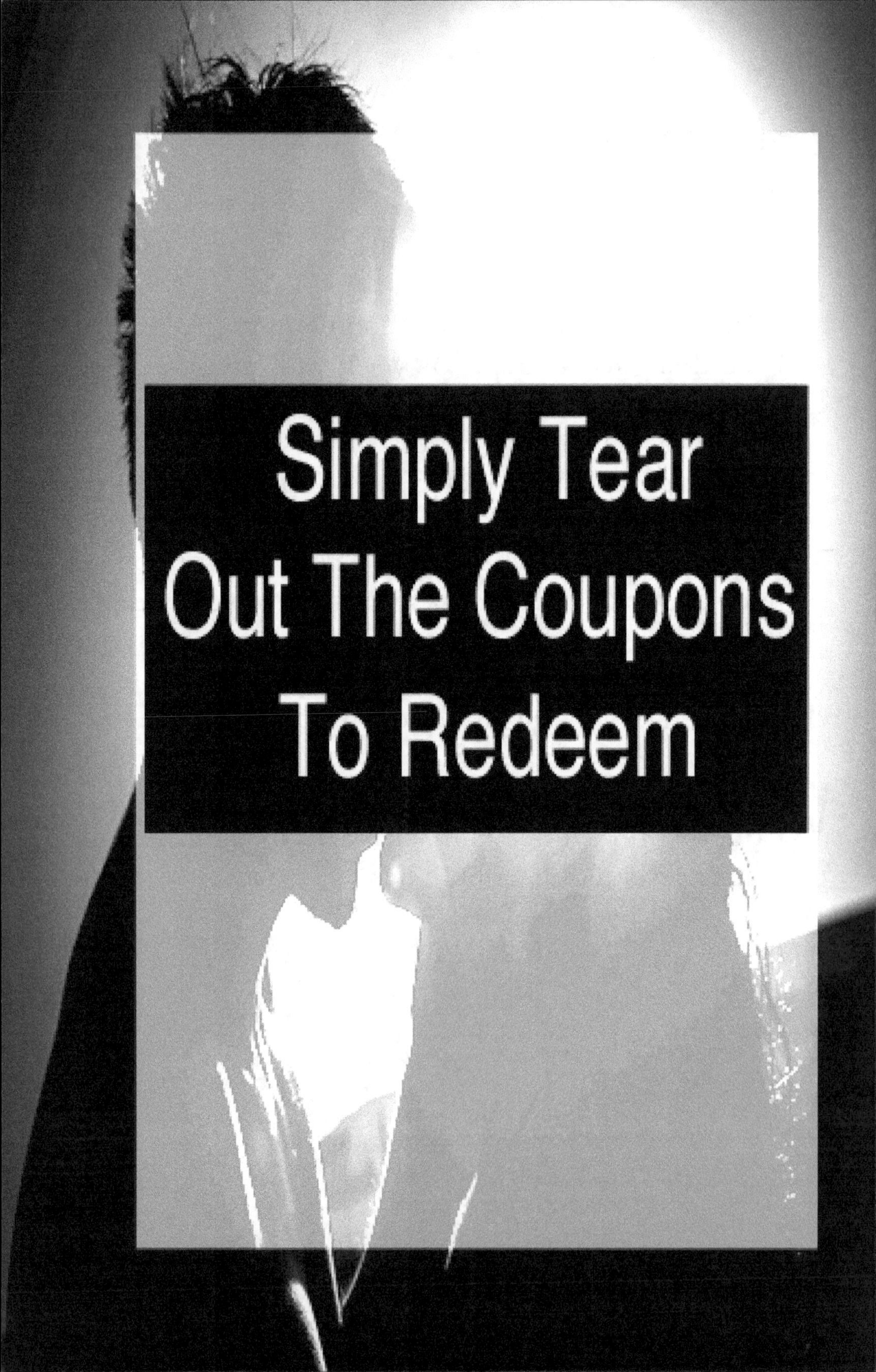
Simply Tear
Out The Coupons
To Redeem

Goal:

Go to the Gym 5 Times A Week For One Month doing intense Fitness Training..

Reward:

I will Pleasure you orally every day at least twice for one entire week.

If You Fail:

You will give me a blowjob Twice a day for one week.

Backside
Of
Coupon

Goal:

Lose five pounds in a week

Reward:

I will be your sex slave
for an entire day.

If You Fail:

You will be my sex slave
for an enire day.

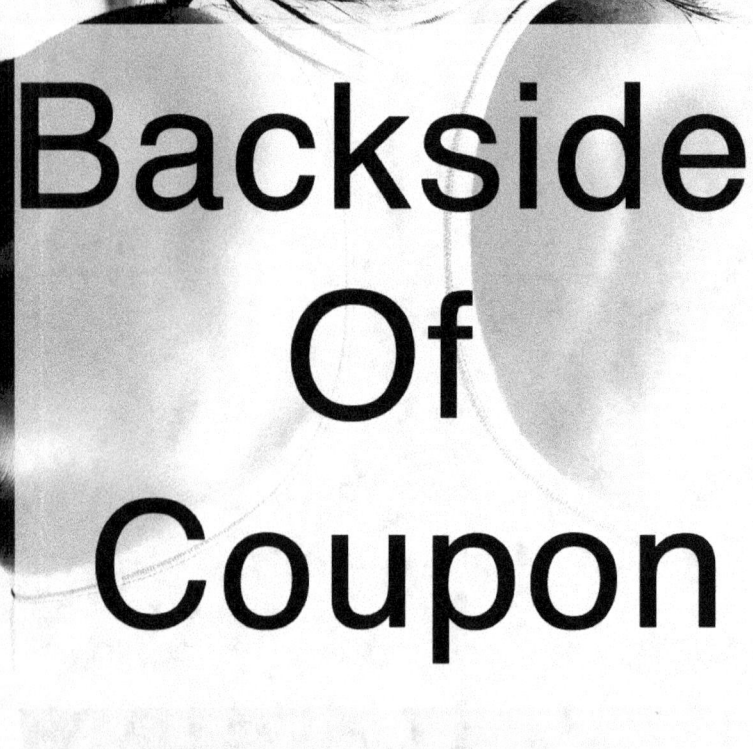

Goal:

Run a 5K Marathon

Reward:

I will clean the house,
do the dishes, and
any other chore, plus your
favorite sex possition.

If You Fail:

You must give me a lap dance
and be tied up while i do you
doggystyle.

Backside
Of
Coupon

Goal:

Stick to your diet protocal for 6 weeks. If you don't have one that find one.

Reward:

I will cook you a meal and give you a 30 minute massage with a happy ending.

If You Fail:

I get an hour long massage with A happy ending.

Backside
Of
Coupon

Goal:

Workout with me for an entire month. I give you the workou protocal and you have to do it.

Reward:

You can write down 5 things you want in bed and I will do them for a week.

If You Fail:

I will write down 5 things in bed I want and you must do them for a week.

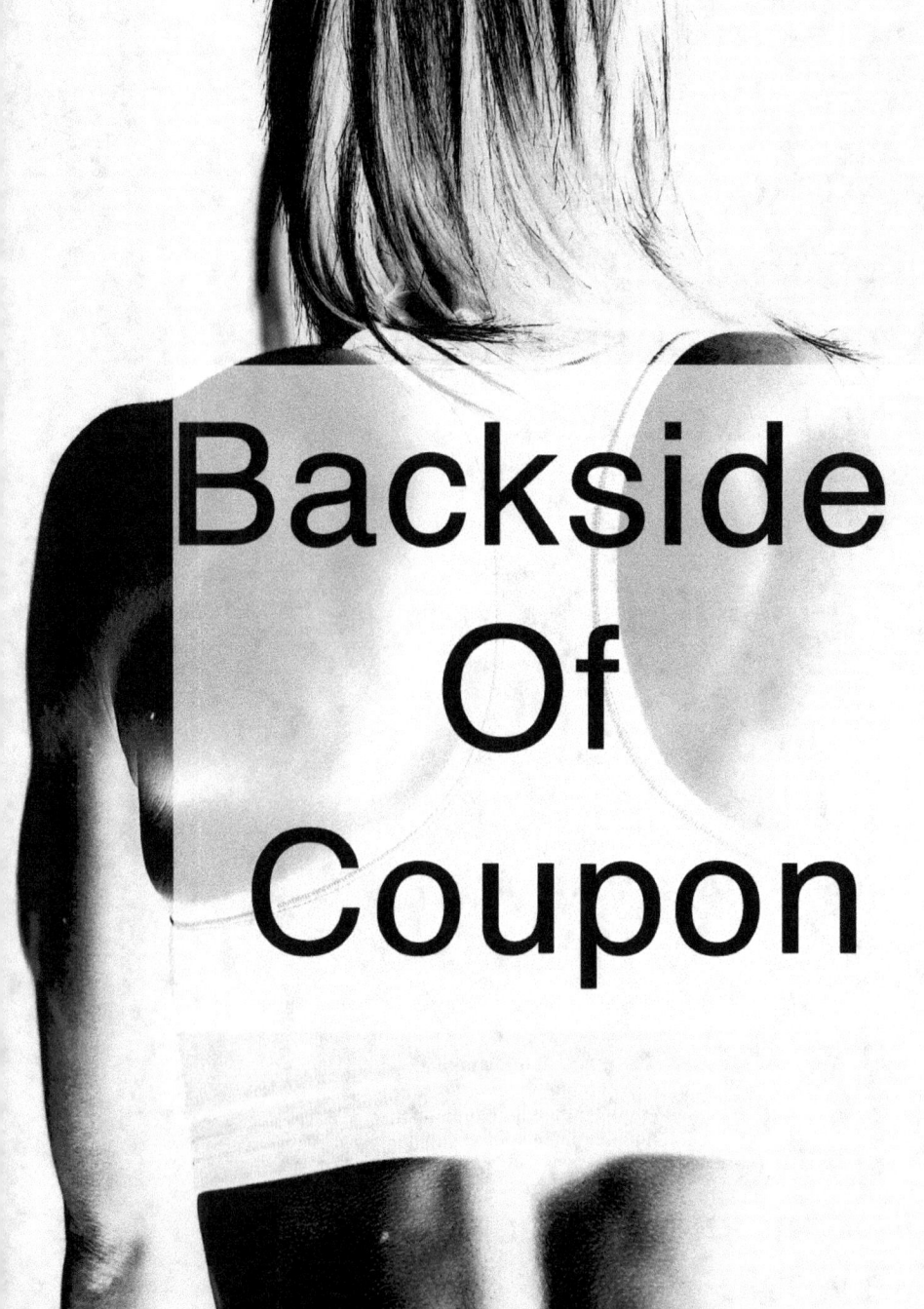

Backside
Of
Coupon

Goal:

You have to lose 10 pounds in one month

Reward:

I will buy you a dress and pleasure you in the shower everyday for a week.

If You Fail:

I will make you give me a blowjob in the shower, while you play with yourself for an entire week.

Backside
Of
Coupon

Goal:

You have to do 1000 squats in one hour. You only get 1 try, and I have to watch and time and make sure you are going all the way down.

Reward:

I will give you one night of romantic dinner, dancing, movie, and whatever you want.

If You Fail:

I want you to give me blowjobs, sex, whatever I want while I play video games, watch movies, for two days.

Backside
Of
Coupon

Those were some fun examples coupons. That you can try out Now you can write in your own goals, rewards, and what will happen if you don't reach your goal.

This could be anything from Spanking, butt play, anal, butt plugs, tied down and vibed all night, etc....

Whatever your into you can do.

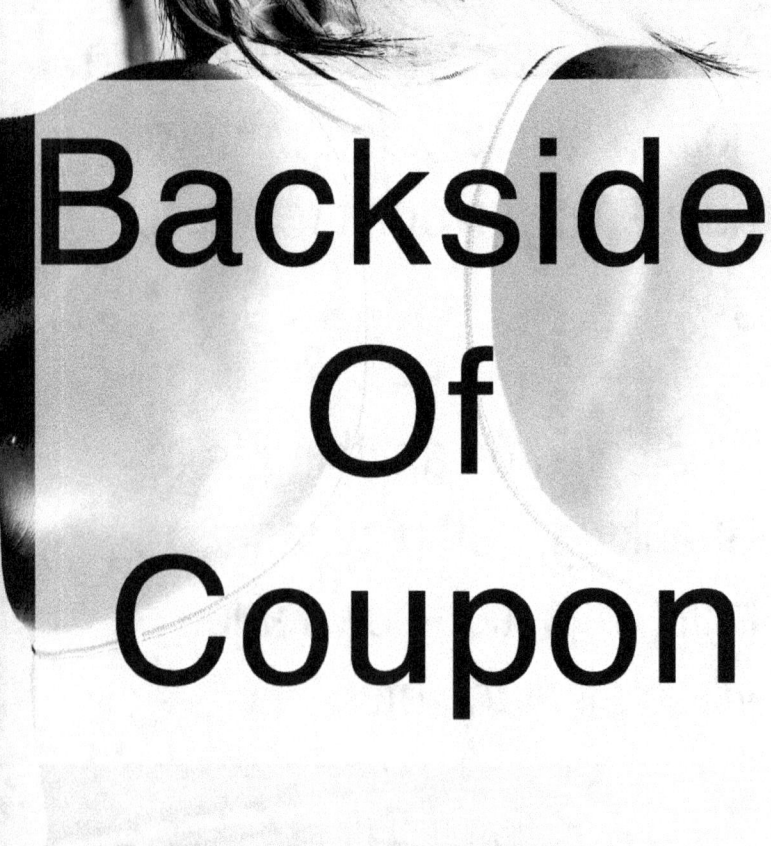

Backside
Of
Coupon

Goal:

_____
_____
_____
_____
_____
_____
_____
_____
_____
_____
_____

Reward:

_____
_____
_____
_____
_____
_____

If You Fail:

_____
_____
_____
_____

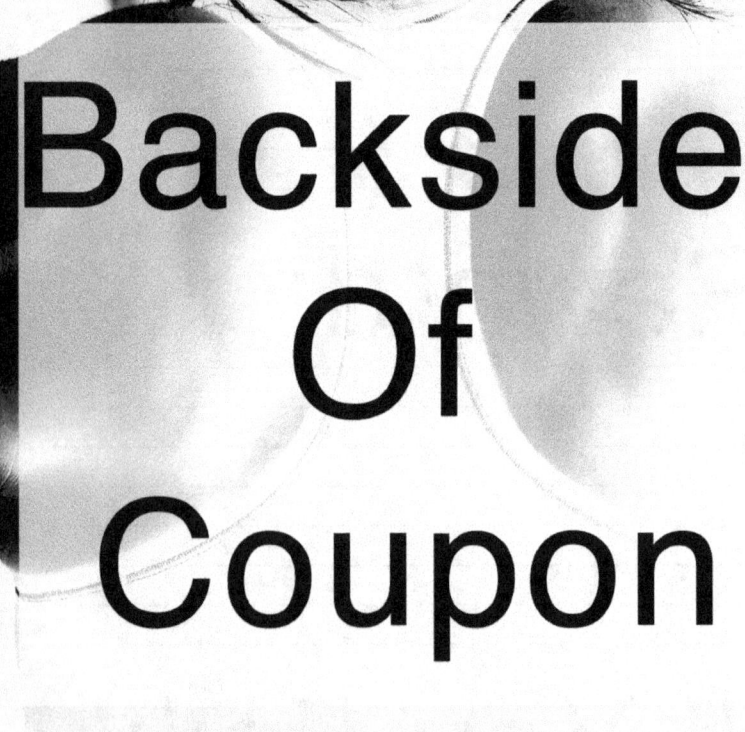

Backside
Of
Coupon

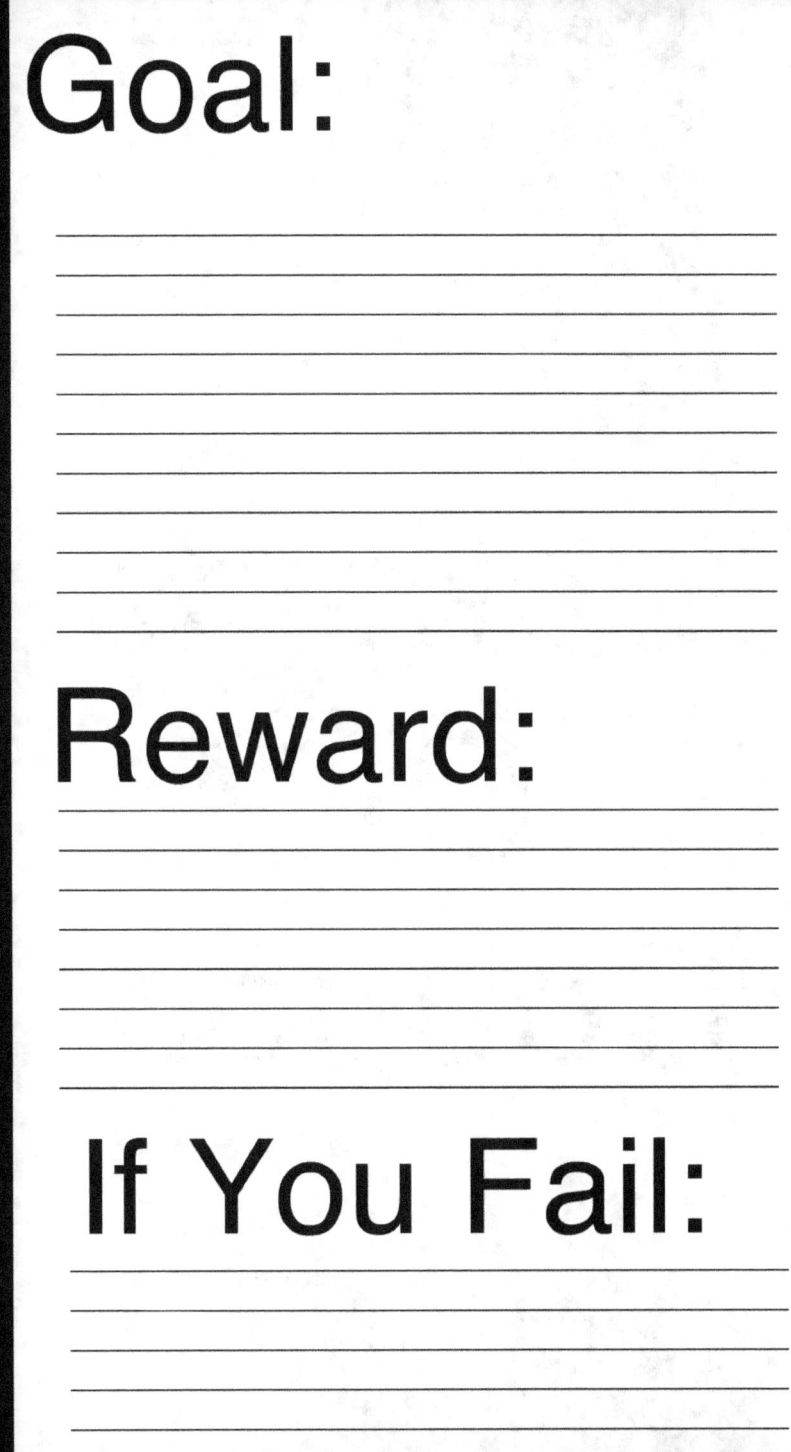

Goal:

_____
_____
_____
_____
_____
_____
_____
_____
_____
_____

Reward:

_____
_____
_____
_____
_____
_____

If You Fail:

_____
_____
_____
_____

Backside
Of
Coupon

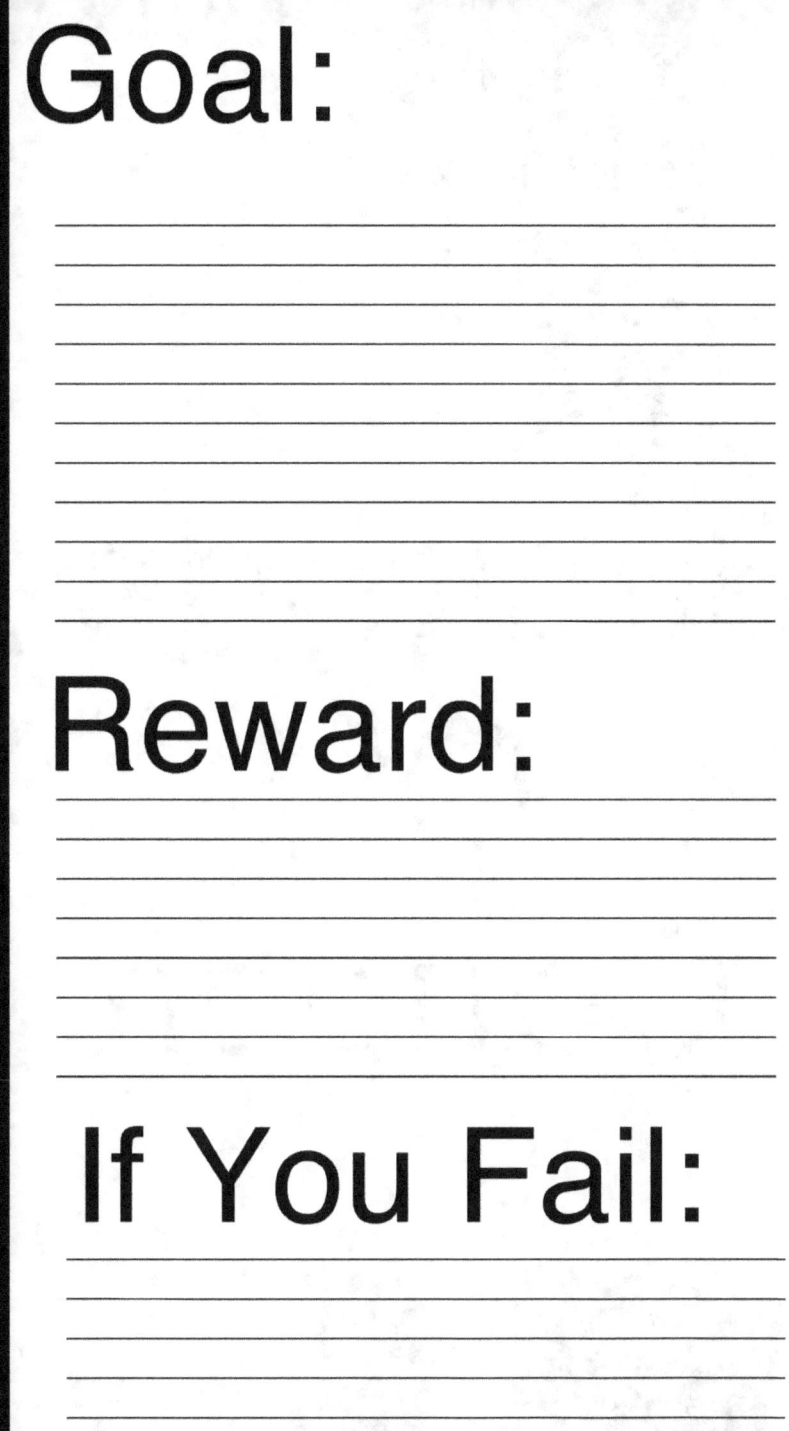

Goal:

_____
_____
_____
_____
_____
_____
_____
_____
_____
_____

Reward:

_____
_____
_____
_____
_____
_____

If You Fail:

_____
_____
_____
_____
_____

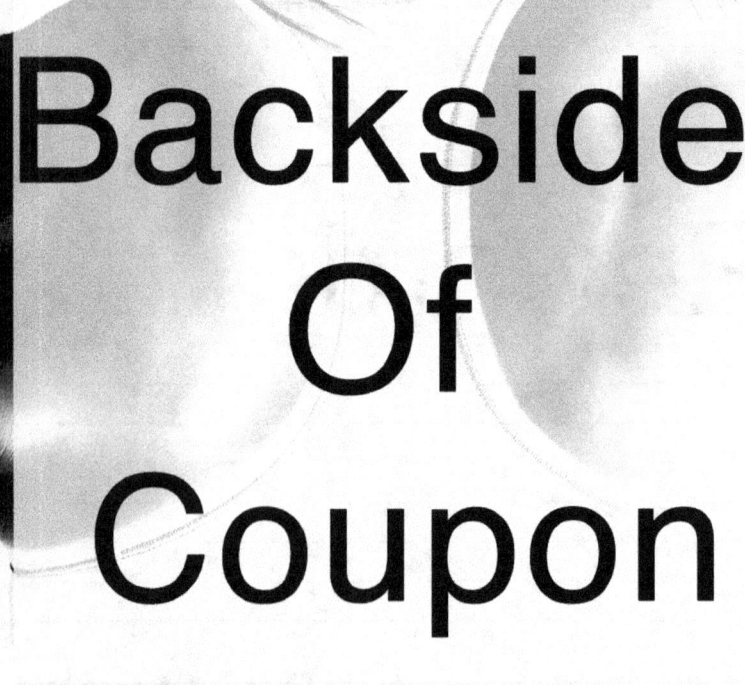

Backside
Of
Coupon

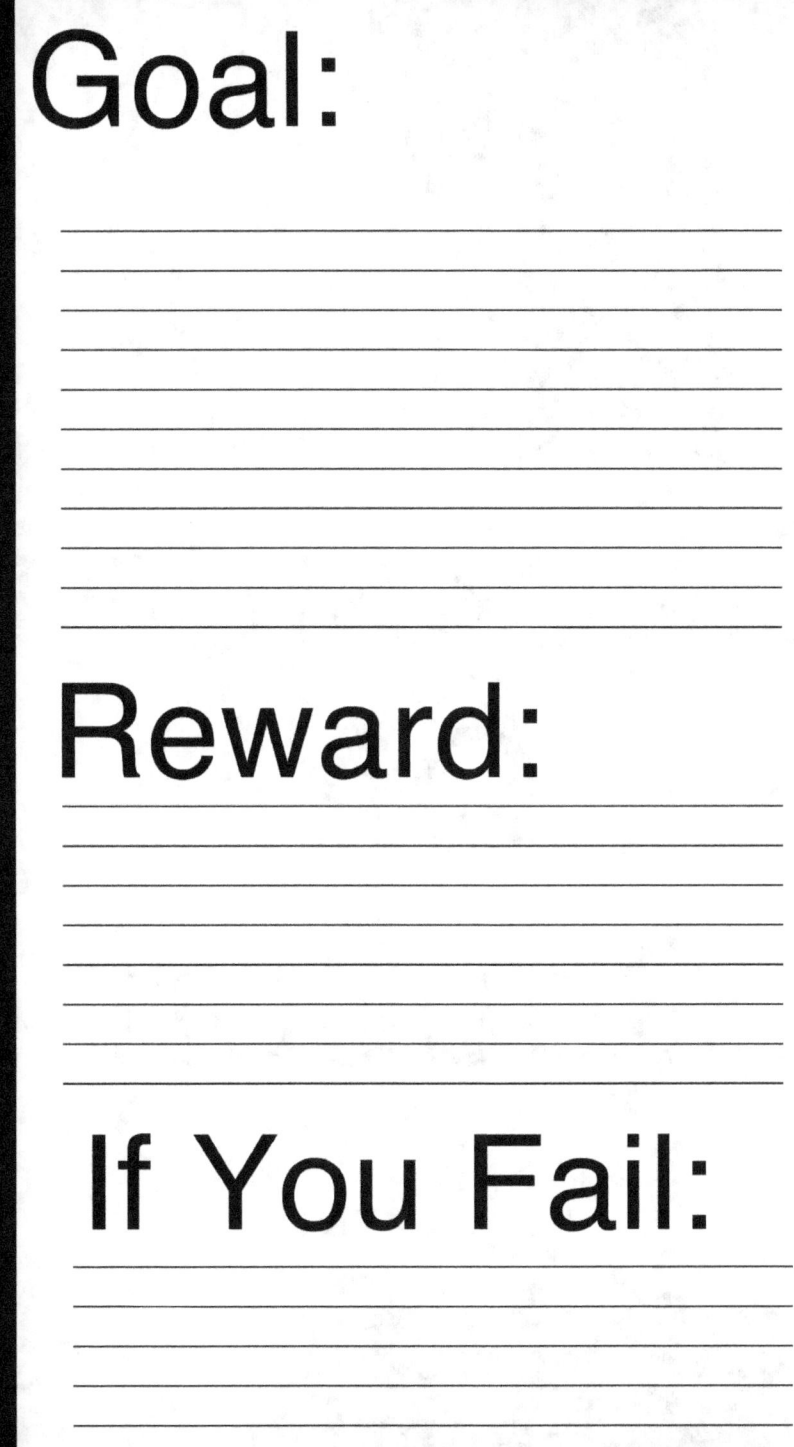

Goal:

_____
_____
_____
_____
_____
_____
_____
_____
_____
_____

Reward:

_____
_____
_____
_____
_____
_____

If You Fail:

_____
_____
_____
_____

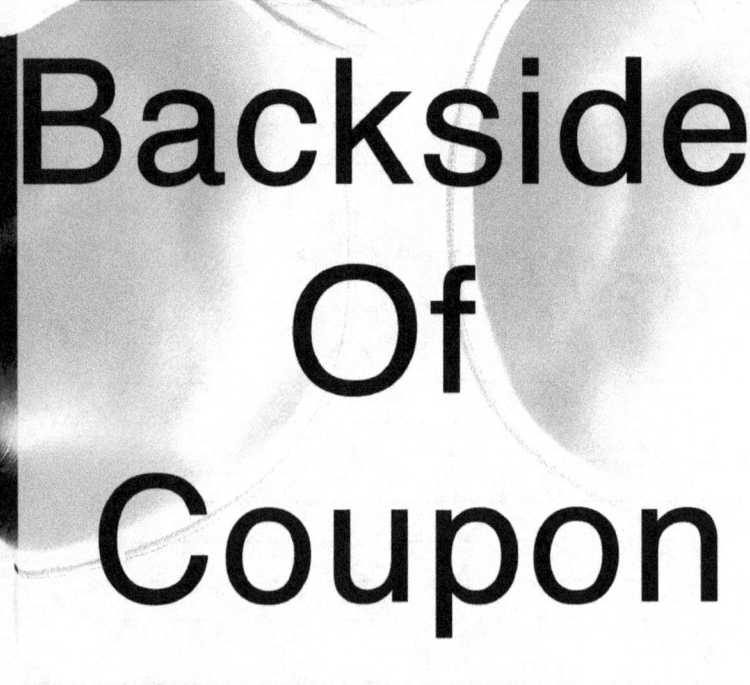

Backside
Of
Coupon

Other Products by J.L. Silver

Valentine Day Sex Coupons

Sex Checks

Sex Vouchers

Sex Coupons

BDSM Coupons

And Many Many More.

www.ingramcontent.com/pod-product-compliance
Lightning Source LLC
Chambersburg PA
CBHW070837310526
45788CB00017B/2027